The Kama Sutra Guide:

Proven Tips For Guaranteed satisfaction and immense pleasure

Disclamer: All photos used in this book, including the cover photo were made available under a Attribution–NonCommercial–ShareAlike 2.0 Generic and sourced from Flickr

Table of Contents

Introduction

Kama Sutra teaches a lot of valuable things, including how to obtain and maintain a satisfying sex life. The art of lovemaking goes beyond the sexual intercourse, allowing you to discover the powerful effect caresses and touches have on you and your partner.

 It provides valuable lessons on foreplay, with both fellatio and cunnilingus techniques that are meant to intensify the pleasure of the upcoming sexual act.

When you start reading about Kama Sutra, it is practically impossible not to feel drawn to its lessons. You are taught that both kissing and embracing your partner can heighten the level of arousal.

Even scratching and biting are presented as part of the lovemaking process, as long as everything is consensual. The main idea is to increase the arousal of your partner to the highest possible level, so as the both of you reach a mind-blowing orgasm.

As you will have the opportunity to read in the chapters that follow, there are many sexual positions to try out and discover as part of the Kama Sutra practice. While some of them are fairly easy, others might prove out to be quite challenging, requiring physical stamina, flexibility and courage.

The sexual positions that are presented as part of this practice encourage the active participation of both partners; this is based on the idea that equal participation guarantees an equal amount of pleasure.

Take your time to read the entire book, discovering how you can use this ancient lovemaking art, in order to satisfy your partner and his/her sexual desires. Learn how to use foreplay to intensify sexual pleasure, resorting to kissing, caressing, holding and embracing.

In this way, you will always keep him/her coming back for more, enjoying satisfying sexual experiences.

Chapter 1 – What is Kama Sutra?

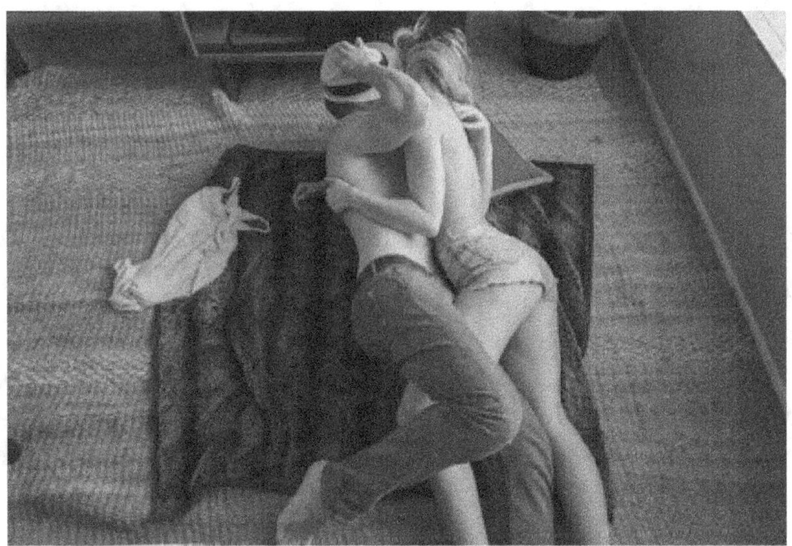

Kama Sutra is an ancient Hindu text, which offers, among other information, practical advice on the art of lovemaking. From this book stems the art of love, one that is based on the pleasures of sensual living.

History tells us that Kama Sutra was written and developed by Nandi, who was the companion of Shiva. It seems that Nandi felt inspired to write Kama Sutra, upon hearing Shiva and his wife, Parvati, making love.

The act of love is widely discussed in the book of Kama Sutra, being split into various methods, which are further divided into a number of sexual positions. In total, we are talking about 64 lovemaking positions, many of them concentrated on the concept of female satisfaction.

The main idea behind this lovemaking art is to strengthen the connection that exists between two people; on one hand, you will engage in sexual intercourse, in order to create the following generation and, on the other hand, you will enjoy giving and receiving both pleasure and variety.

When practiced correctly, this lovemaking art can increase your current level of sexual awareness. Moreover, it can teach you how to develop the proper respect for the sacredness of sexual intercourse. In fact, you are given a lesson even from the name of the practice, as "kama" stands for love, sexual gratification and erotic practice.

As for "sutra", this actually refers to something that allows for everything to stay together. From all of these things, it can be easily suggested that Kama Sutra is the practice that teaches you how to use sexual relations as a way to demonstrate your love to one another.

As you will dive further and discover more on this ancient lovemaking art, you will find out that Kama Sutra is more than sex. It teaches you about the importance of kissing and caressing your partner, so that you develop a connection that goes beyond the physical world.

As for the sexual positions that are presented as part of the Kama Sutra practice, these are meant to enhance the connection between a man and a woman as well.

With Kama Sutra, you may start at a physical level but, soon, you will be able to discover a deeper connection with your partner.

Many people discover the art of love that is Kama Sutra when they are at a point in their lives when they need something more. They acknowledge that their partner is no longer as interesting as it used to be, seeking out answers.

With the practice of Kama Sutra, one has the opportunity to re-discover his/her partner, trying out new things and enjoying the creative aspect of sexual experiences. Kama Sutra is the kind of practice that allows for sexual attraction to be maintained, including a number of erotic experiences that are definitely worth trying.

Kama Sutra will teach you that you need to create a sacred space for lovemaking, in order to enjoy the experience to the fullest. It will help you to take sexual intercourse to a whole new level, going from a simple physical experience to a sensual and incredibly rewarding form of art. As you will proceed through discovering the art of love, you will go from normal intercourse to energy sex, one that is based on a deep connection.

The practice of Kama Sutra allows you to become a better lover, stimulating your emotions and inner energy at the same time. When you practice this form of lovemaking, you have the opportunity to demonstrate genuine love to your partner, whether it is through touching, rubbing or pressing your bodies together. As for the sexual positions, these are guaranteed to open your eyes, allowing you to gain a completely new perspective on life.

Chapter 2 – How can Kama Sutra benefit your sex life?

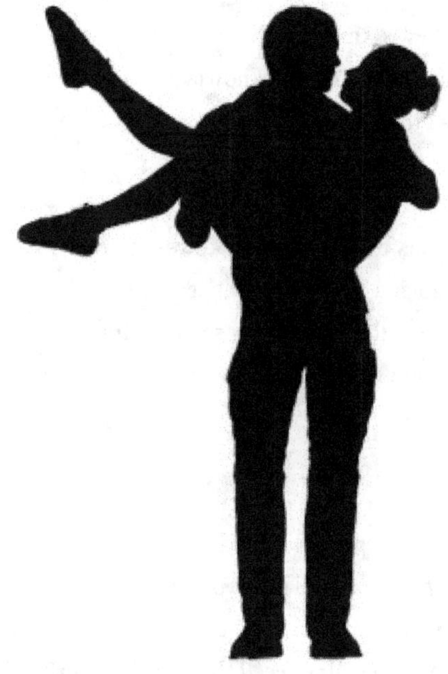

The regular practice of Kama Sutra can make you feel more comfortable with your own sexuality, increasing your appetite for new experiences. Basically, after you master the genuine art of lovemaking, you will be more inclined to seek out sexual pleasures.

Kama Sutra will teach you to go from sex to lovemaking, as a unique form of art; moreover, you will learn how to be closer to your partner, finally feeling like your life is balanced.

Perhaps the most important benefit to consider is the lack of monotony. Kama Sutra will challenge you to try out a number of different positions, thus enhancing your sex life.

For long-term couples, in which routine can lead to boredom in the bedroom, the sexual positions included in this practice can rekindle the flame of passion. When you try something new, it is highly likely that you will gain more enjoyment from the lovemaking process.

The great thing about Kama Sutra is that it can help in all areas involved in the lovemaking process, including when it comes to preparation and foreplay.

It can generate a close connection between partners during the actual intercourse, as well as during the after play. As you try out the different sexual positions, you will be able to acknowledge the needs of your partner in a more efficient manner, both physically and mentally.

For a lot of people, sexual intercourse is just a mechanical act, without intimacy and deep connections being part of the process. Kama Sutra teaches that you can fulfill the needs of the partner, enjoying yourself at the same time. And it does not concern solely the sexual intercourse but everything that surrounds it.

For example, you are taught that you can set the mood for a nice sexual experience by lighting candles or using fabrics to hide rough corners. It teaches you how to prepare for sexual intercourse by showering and shaving, highlighting the importance of sensual touches during the foreplay phase.

The practice of Kama Sutra can bring two partners closer than ever. This is because you will have the opportunity to try out both easy and challenging positions.

As you will give these new positions a chance, you will most likely make a mistake, something which can be turned into a fun and stimulating experience. Trying to figure the logistics together, you will bond without even being aware of what is actually happening.

No matter if you are a prude or not, Kama Sutra teaches you to get out of your comfort zone. It highlights the importance of oral sex, with plenty of techniques to try out for both fellatio and cunnilingus.

On one hand, your partner will be aroused, seeing that you are willing to try out new things and forget about your usual routine. Second, they will reach the highest peaks of pleasure, the two of you enjoying a fantastic foreplay together. When the foreplay is as amazing as described, you can only imagine how great the sexual intercourse is going to be.

When you engage in the art of lovemaking, you are also gain more confidence in your own abilities. However, you must not forget that Kama Sutra is all about active participation, involving both sexes in an equal manner.

Many of the sexual positions that you are going to try out will require that both partners are active; this is going to be a challenge, as you will have to switch from your regular positions to something completely new. However, when you will see how much pleasure you are experiencing, you will understand that it was all worth it.

The sexual positions included in the practice of Kama Sutra do not encourage the woman to be a passive receiver, but rather an active participant to the sexual act. There are many positions that are based on the equal involvement of the partners, generating an equal amount of pleasure.

The variety offered is one of the main reasons people turn to this lovemaking practice; moreover, one can enjoy new sexual positions, without worrying about his/her body shape or size.

The practice of Kama Sutra will teach you another important lesson and that is that touch does matter. As the years go by, couples tend to concentrate less on touch and more on the sexual act per say.

Well, touch does matter and this is not valid only for the sexual intercourse; the more partners touch one another, the higher the chance to experience arousing sensations. Touch is extremely sensual and it can increase the intensity of the sexual experience, starting from the actual foreplay and until the very end.

Kama Sutra will take you from a monotonous and mechanical sex life to something amazing. The new sexual positions, the constant touching and caressing, all of these things are going to turn you into a new person.

Moreover, you will finally be able to understand that there is stronger method of conveying your emotions than through touch. Last, but not least, you will have the opportunity to re-discover the fact that sex is fun. You will experiment, having fun with your partner and forgetting all about your previous boring, mechanical sessions in the bedroom.

Chapter 3 – Kama Sutra foreplay techniques

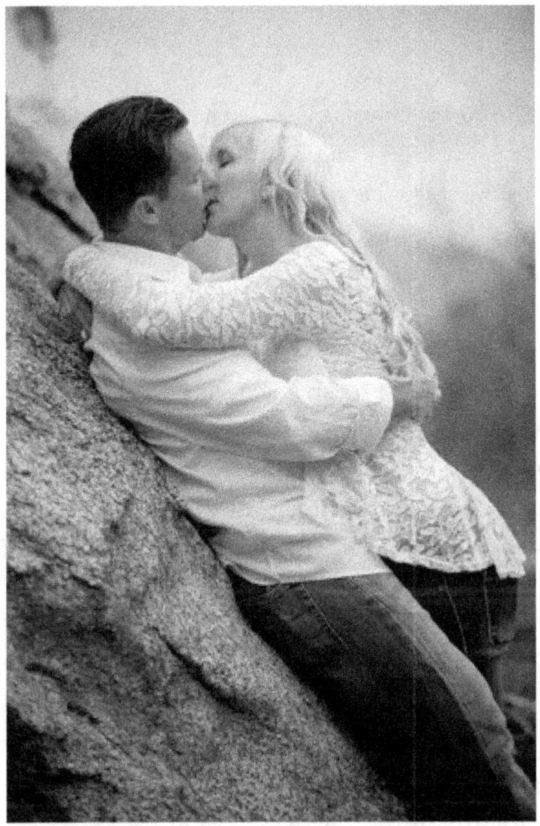

A successful sexual experience is guaranteed by a generous foreplay, this is one of the most important lessons that Kama Sutra teaches us. Once you focus on increasing your partner's sexual arousal, either through simple kissing or through oral sex, you will be one step closer to a passionate lovemaking experience.

Let us find more information on the different techniques that are recommended for foreplay by Kama Sutra practitioners.

Kissing

Even the simplest of kisses can provide your partner with immense pleasure, so you can definitely consider such practices as suitable for the foreplay phase. Kissing brings pleasure to both partners, allowing you to prepare for the actual sexual intercourse. The good news is that kissing can be continued during the intercourse, guaranteeing not only intimacy but also prolonged pleasure.

The bent kiss is deeply intimate, with the two lovers bending their heads toward each other. You can also try the turned kiss, holding your lover by his/her chin, before performing the actual kiss. This is considered a more intense form of kissing, generating a higher level of arousal. The straight kiss tells the partner what you are thinking of in a straightforward manner, being however intimate and powerful.

The clasping kiss occurs when you are talking your partner's lips between your own, increasing the sexual tension between you without any effort. Last, but not least, you have the fighting of the tongue, in which you will use your tongue to touch not only the tongue but also the palate and teeth of your partner.

This is considered indeed the most passionate form of kissing, being perfect for a heated sexual experience.

Cunnilingus techniques (licking of the rose petals)

Women take immense pleasure from oral sex but, with the passing of time, your routine can become monotonous and less stimulating. Kama Sutra teaches a wide range of cunnilingus techniques, allowing you to bring a lot of pleasure to your partner.

One of the most important cunnilingus techniques is known as the "quivering kiss". In this technique, you will have to use your fingertips, in order to bring the labia close together. Then, you will have to kiss them, as if you were kissing your partner's actual lips.

Another technique is presented as the "circling tongue", being based on you using your tongue to gently penetrate the vagina. While your tongue performs circling motions, make sure to be extremely gentle, as the interior of the vagina can be pretty sensitive. Also, it might be a good idea to shave, in order to reduce the risk of irritation down there.

The "tongue massage" is a technique that requires a slow penetration of the vagina, with the tongue resting a moment before the actual entering. The rhythm is extremely important in this technique and the sexual pleasure is guaranteed, as long as you apply pressure in different areas, without resting on one in particular.

The "sucked" technique requires that you fasten your lips to the labia, performing deep kisses on your partner. Basically, you will suck hard at the clitoris, hence the name of the technique.

A similar technique is the one that is known as "sucked up"; for this technique, you will have to lift the buttocks of your partner, using your tongue to stimulate the entrance of the vagina. You will then create a suction motion, pleasing your partner in a unique and novel way.

The "stirring" technique is based on the idea of mutual cooperation between the two partners. While the woman opens her thighs and thus provides the partner with better access to her secret parts, the man uses his tongue to penetrate the vagina and performs stirring motions.

The "sucked hard" technique is innovative to say the least and may be a little bit challenging for some people. While your partner rests her feet on your shoulders, you will grab her by the waist, sucking hard on the clitoris.

Last, but not least, you have the "crow" technique, which is actually the original version of the 69 position. You and your partner will have to lie side by side, kissing each other's intimate areas and enjoying the immense pleasure of the foreplay phase.

Fellatio techniques (sucking a mango fruit)

Caressing your partner's intimate area can bring a lot of pleasure to him, preparing the terrain for the exciting moment of sexual intercourse. While there are many techniques available, you have to remember that the penis is sensitive and you have to be gentle when performing oral sex.

A good starting technique is the one that involves licking the penis. Basically, you have to imagine that the penis is an ice cream cone and lick it as such. Make sure to hold the base with one hand, performing licking motions on the sides of the penis, in an alternate manner and in an upward direction.

The penis has a lot of sensitive points, this being the reason why you can consider the "butterfly flick". For this technique, you will have to hold the penis at the base with one hand, making sure that you flick the tongue on the penile ridge. As for the "nominal congress", this involves taking the penis in your hand and placing it between your lips. Then, all you have to do is move it gently around the mouth, making sure to avoid any harsh teeth contact.

"Biting the sides" is another interesting fellatio technique, one that definitely can be used for increasing the heat of passion between two partners. You can start by covering the penis head with the fingertips, then using your teeth to gently nibble on the sides.

Once again, it should be mentioned that you have to be gentle, otherwise the whole experience is going to be painful and not at all pleasurable.

If you want to increase your partner's arousal even more, you have to give the "pressing inside" technique a try. First of all, take the penis into the mouth and, then, use your lips to apply pressure.

Repeat the process for extended pleasure. As for the "pressing outside" technique, this requires that you press the lips against the end of the penis. Then, kiss the penis, as it comes out of your mouth, using plenty of saliva for lubrication purposes.

The "rubbing" technique involves kissing the penis on its entire surface. Then, use your tongue to lick it; when you will reach the end of the penis, make sure to perform rubbing motions for intense pleasure. You can then continue with the "kissing" technique, using your lips to kiss the tip of the penis, as if you were kissing his lower lip.

One of the most famous fellatio techniques that is part of the Kama Sutra practice is known as "sucking a mango fruit". In order to perform this technique, you will have to take the penis into your mouth, at approximately half way. For the next step, you will have to apply vigorous sucking motions, making sure to avoid the teeth contact.

Last, but not least, you have the "swallowing up" technique, in which you will practically try to take the whole length of the penis inside your mouth. This can be extremely stimulating for your partner, so make sure you give it a try.

Chapter 4 – Kama Sutra lovemaking positions

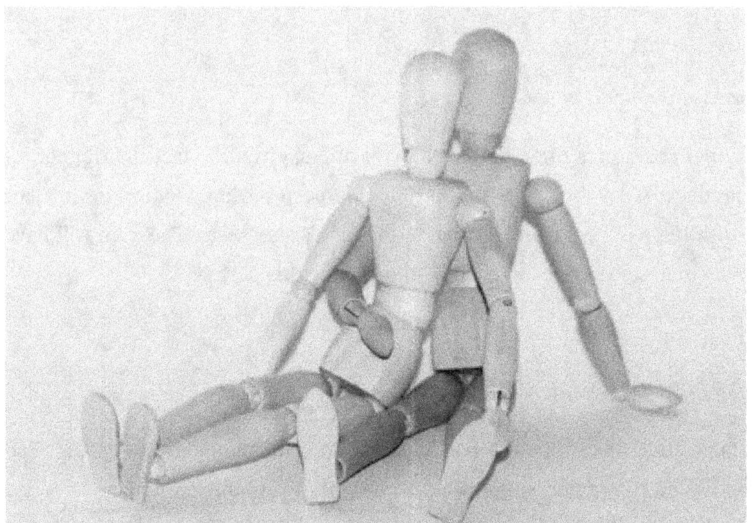

Once you have moved past the foreplay phase, it is time to engage in some serious lovemaking. There are numerous Kama Sutra sexual positions for you to try out, rekindling the flame of passion between you and your partner. These sexual positions are meant to eliminate monotony and boredom from the bedroom, allowing yourself to enjoy a beautiful and satisfying sexual experience.

Yawning sexual position

The man stands on his knees, touching hands with the partner, who lies on her back. The woman keeps her legs in the air, pressing them into the partner's hips for more pleasure.

The variant yawning position

This sexual position is often preferred by partners, given the fact that it guarantees the deepest level of penetration. For this position, the woman lies on her back, with the feet in the air, resting on the man's shoulders. The man will have the inside of his elbows nestled behind the knees of his partner.

The widely opened position

For this position, the woman lies on her back, with the thighs widely spread. The partner lies on top of her, supporting the weight of his body on his hands. As he prepares to enter the kingdom of love, the woman raises her pelvis and meets her partner halfway.

Wife of Indra position

This position is recommended for those with limber bodies, as it requires some flexibility. The woman lies on her back, with her knees tucked in, so that they rest on her breasts. This position is known in the Kama Sutra book as one of the most complex, given the fact that it allows for the maximum penetration of the vagina. The man is on his knees, using the body of the partner for support.

Clasping position

For this position, the man lies on his back, with the partner being on top. This is known as an intimate position, due to the fact that the limbs of both partners are intertwined.

Side-by-side clasping position

The starting position is with both partners on their sides, looking each other into the eyes. It is recommended that the man lies on the left side, while the woman is on her right side. The intertwining of the limbs creates a feeling of intimacy as in the above-mentioned position.

Indian handstand position

When it comes to the Indian handstand position, the woman lies on her back, with the thighs spread apart. One leg might be flexed and the other one extended. The man will penetrate the woman from the lateral side, keeping both knees flexed.

The lotus blossom position

For this position, the man will sit in a cross-legged position. As for the woman, she will sit on her partner, wrapping her legs around his waist. The man will guide the movements of his partner, the hands resting on her hips. He might also caress her breasts and touch her bottom for more pleasure.

The eagle position

The man will kneel in front the partner, most commonly at the edge of the bed. The woman lies on her back, with the legs spread apart. The man will grab the woman by the ankles, the two of them enjoying the deep and satisfying penetration that such a position guarantees. Placing a pillow under the woman might enhance the pleasure of this position.

The rider position

If you are feeling adventurous, you can give the rider position a try. For this position, the man lies on his back. The woman rides her partner but with her back at the partner. She may lean forward, in order to maintain her balance and also for more pleasure.

The amazon position

For this position, the man will sit comfortably on a chair of his choice. The woman will come and sit down on him, facing in a forward direction. This position is highly stimulating, allowing the woman to reach orgasm in a more facile manner.

The peg position

The man is going to lie on his side for this position. The woman will be on her side as well, but the head will be on the opposite part, facing the feet of the partner. The woman practically embraces the feet of her partner, while he enters into her kingdom of love.

The column position

For this position, both partners are standing, so physical stamina is more than required. The woman will be with her back to the partner, enjoying the deep penetration. The arms of both partners can be intertwined for the maintenance of proper balance.

Bandoleer position

The woman lies on her back, with her head resting on a pillow and the knees bent, toward the chest (but not resting on it). The man will kneel in front of his partner, allowing the woman to place her feet on his chest.

The bridge position

This is indeed one of the most challenging lovemaking positions, requiring a lot of flexibility and physical resistance on behalf of the man. While he maintains the bridge-like position, the woman will practically ride him, supporting her hands on his body.

The grip position

The woman lies on her back, the arms resting on the lateral sides of the body. The man stands on all fours, while the woman raises her pelvis in order to meet his partner. In order to make the position more comfortable, you can place a cushion under the woman's bottom.

Afternoon delight position

For this position, the man lies on his side, using his hand to support the head. The woman lies on her back as well, on a perpendicular axe in comparison to the man. This position does not require too much effort and it is highly recommended after a long lovemaking session.

The slide position

The man lies on his back, while the woman lies on him, with the legs held close one to the other. While the man enters into her kingdom of love, she will rub up and down his body (hence the name of the position).

The standing clasp position

For this position, the man stands upright, while the woman wraps her legs around his waist. This position requires physical stamina from the man, as he will have to support his partner completely. If you are looking to obtain more support and enjoy a deeper penetration, you can help your partner rest with her back against a wall.

The glowing juniper position

The woman lies on her back, the legs being spread apart and the knees slightly bent. The man will have to slide between her legs, lifting her hips just a little bit, in order to facilitate the penetration process. The experience can be made more intimate, as the man lifts his partner and caresses or kisses her abdomen.

The seated ball position

For this position, the woman will have to adopt a crouched posture. The man is found in a half-sitting position, from which he will attempt to penetrate his partner (from behind). The woman is in control of the movement, using her heels to gently rock back and forth. The man can give the woman more pleasure by kissing her back.

The curled angel position

The woman will adopt a curled up position, drawing her knees to the chest. The man will spoon his partner, taking advantage of the fairly easy penetration. The great advantage of this position is that the man can stimulate his partner, caressing her breasts or playing with her clitoris.

The perch position

For this position, the man sits on a chair, taking his partner on his lap. The woman has her back at the partner. Using the physical force of her legs, she will handle the movements of the sexual act. As for the partner, he will use his hands to either caress the breasts or clitoris of his partner. Leaning in a forward direction will facilitate the penetration process.

Chapter 5 – Kama Sutra caresses and sensual touching

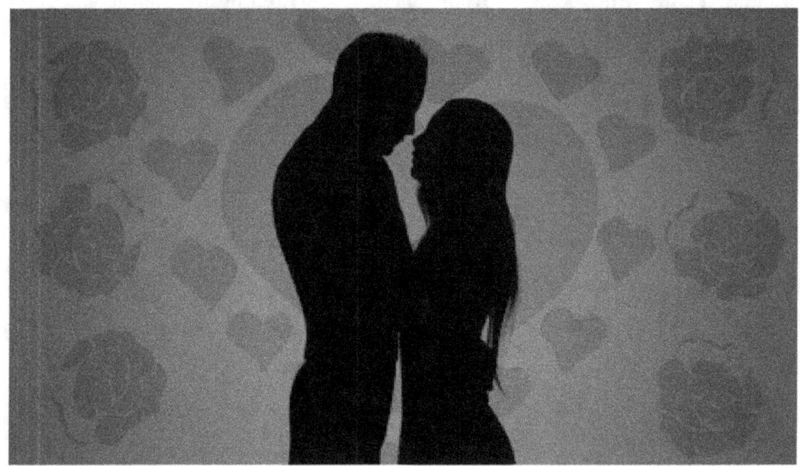

The caresses and sensual touches that are included in the practice of Kama Sutra can bring partners closer together. For couples who have been together for a long period of time, it is through such practices that they are able to restore the flame of passion and re-discover one another.

Embraces of Kama Sutra

The "touching embrace" refers to a man or a woman that uses his or her body, in order to touch the partner. The "rubbing embrace" refers to couples that rub their bodies one against the other.

As for the "pressing embrace", this refers to pressing the partner's body against a wall. Other forms of embraces that can be tried out include the "piercing embrace", the "embrace of the thighs" and the "embrace of the breasts".

Kama Sutra embraces are simple to practice, yet they have a multitude of benefits to offer to both partners. They can be used to relax the body and clear the mind, in preparation for a satisfying lovemaking session. On the other hand, an embrace can bring partners closer together, allowing them to touch their intimate areas and experience arousal.

Bathing and mutual cleansing

Couples who bathe or shower together enjoy a higher level of intimacy, not to mention that such rituals can facilitate a stimulating sexual experience. Allow yourself the luxury of spending time being caressed by your partner, while the hot water relaxes and arouses your body at the same time. Use plenty of soap, as this will facilitate the gliding of the hands across the skin, increasing the level of arousal for both you and your partner.

Scratching and biting

The practice of Kama Sutra can help you bring out your passionate side, with actions such as scratching and biting being part of the lovemaking process. When one expresses his/her passion through such actions, monotony and routine are eliminated from the start. The one thing you have to make sure is that your partner finds these things pleasurable as well. Consider these as marks of passion but always stay within the limits you have established together.

Hair play

Women can enjoy immense pleasure when their partners play with their hair. When the man caresses the woman and strokes her hair, the level of arousal is heightened and a satisfying sexual experience is guaranteed. As for the woman, she can actually use her long hair to arouse her partner; she can caress his entire body, concentrating on the penis as well.

Hair play can bring out sexual desire in both partners but it is important to have shiny and clean hair. The man has to be feel himself drawn to his partner's hair, in order to enjoy the whole experience. A highly stimulating experience can be when partners run their fingers through each other's hair at the same time. Brushing your partner's hair or performing a scalp massage can heighten arousal as well.

Conclusion

If you want to bring passion back to the bedroom, you will give Kama Sutra a try. All you have to do is keep an open mind and try the things that have been suggested in this book. Soon, both you and your partner will enjoy a highly satisfying sexual experience, feeling closer to one another than ever.

The more you will explore each other's desires, the better your relationship is going to be. No more routine or monotony to worry about. Just the feeling of closeness, brought on by the constant touching and caressing that Kama Sutra entails.

The sexual positions that are recommended as part of the Kama Sutra practice are meant to take you out of your comfort zone. You will finally take your sexuality to a whole new level, as you will try new things and discover your partner from a unique perspective.

In the end, all of these new experiences are going to help you build a more intimate relationship with your partner, one that will stand the test of time. Enjoy the immense pleasure that the practices of Kama Sutra bring, not forgetting that equal participation guarantees an equal amount of satisfaction.

FREE Bonus Reminder

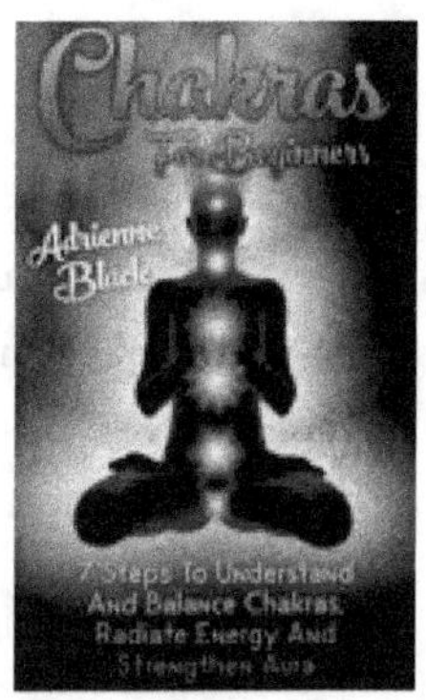

If you have not grabbed it yet, please go ahead and download your special bonus E book *"Chakras for Beginners. 7 Steps To Understand And Balance Chakras, Radiate Energy, And Strengthen Aura"*.

Simply Click the Button Below

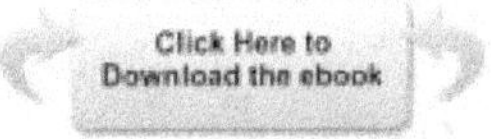

OR **Go to This Page**

http://lifehacksworld.com/free

BONUS #2: More Free & Discounted Books

Do you want to receive more Free & Discounted Books?

We have a mailing list where we send out our new Books when they go free or with a discount on Kindle. Click on the link below to sign up for Free & Discount Book Promotions.

=> Sign Up for Free & Discount Book Promotions <=

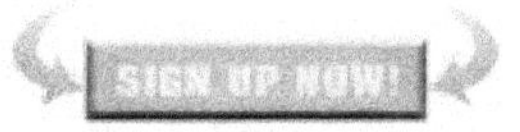

OR Go to this URL

http://zbit.ly/1WBb1Ek